THE LONG GOODBYE

by

Patricia L. Beckler

Blessings!
Pat Beckler

Ideas into Books®
WESTVIEW
Kingston Springs, Tennessee

Ideas into Books® W E S T V I E W
P.O. Box 605
Kingston Springs, TN 37082
www.publishedbywestview.com

ISBN 978-1-62880-088-3

First edition, September 2015

The author gratefully acknowledges permission to reprint: Hymn of Promise © 1986, Hope Publishing Company, Carol Stream, IL. All rights reserved. Used by permission.

Good faith efforts have been made to trace copyrights on materials included in this publication. If any copyrighted material has been included without permission and due acknowledgment, proper credit will be inserted in future printings after notice has been received.

Printed in the United States of America on acid free paper.

A tribute to my husband
John D. Beckler
December 20, 1932--September 13, 2010

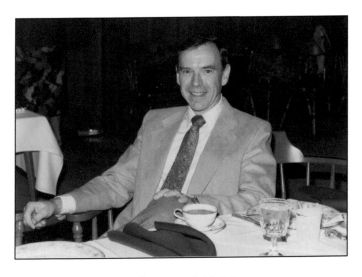

John around 1984

Death leaves a heartache
no one can heal.
Love leaves a memory
no one can steal.

From a headstone in Ireland

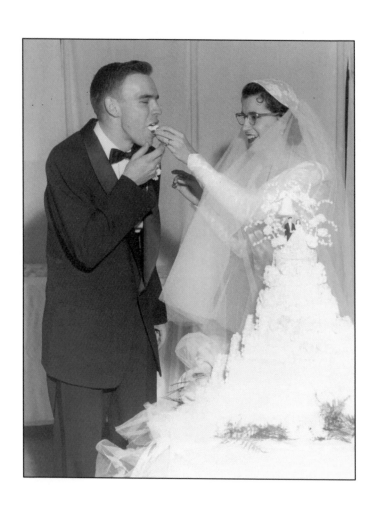

December 22, 1956, Nashville, Tennessee

TABLE OF CONTENTS

ACKNOWLEDGMENTS

Other than my faith, the aspect of my life for which I am most grateful is to have loved and been loved by John Beckler. My deepest sadness during his illness was the knowledge that he was losing touch with our precious family—all those memories, gone. Although I have lost John, our daughters, Cheryl and Celia, and their families continue to be a joy and enrich my life more than I can say. This record is primarily for them, but it is also for those dear and close friends who knew of this journey and walked it with us as much as possible. You know who you are. In addition, I would like to think that our story might be helpful for others who are saying their own Good-bye's.

Most writers include in their acknowledgements, "This book would not have been written without…." True for me, this book would never have happened without the gentle urging of a close Wildewood Downs neighbor and good friend, Dr. O'Neill Barrett, Jr. As we shared life's experiences over many cups of tea, I would relate some episode, several included in this book,

O'Neill would say, "Pat, you need to write that down." Sure thing! In my spare time!

As a few years have gone by, a number of the episodes I've included have taken permanent shape in my mind. So that, at this point, much of the book has almost written itself. I just sat at the computer. Thank you, O'Neill, also for being my major proofreader/editor.

I wish also to thank O'Neill's daughter, Deborah Clements, who a few days ago sat and read aloud to me significant portions of this book. I realized I had truly written what I wanted to say and that the length, short, was correct. Thank you, Deb.

My thanks must also include three special friends who took the time to read the text and to make valuable comments: Ellen Dukes, Jean Hein, and Bonnie Mullis. Thank you, ladies!

Lastly, a word of appreciation to Mary Catharine Nelson, owner of *Ideas into Books*® Westview, for being the best publisher on the planet.

Patricia Beckler
June 30, 2015

THE LONG GOOD-BYE

INTRODUCTION

Why would anyone wish to write a book about some dreadful disease? Especially one as common today as dementia in its many forms. I'm not drawn to read stories about families and their loved ones who have traveled this path. Yet, here I am, preparing to create this written record of how our family lived our story. Our two daughters and their husbands know the story. Our five grandchildren have grown up as we have lived our story. I wish our five precious great-grandchildren (number six due in December) to have some understanding of this gentle man they never knew, to have some sense of his goodness, his intelligence and the steps he took to protect and provide for me since he clearly would not be able to do that for long. Yet...it took fourteen years to tell our story.

In August, 2003, Senior Primary Care asked me to participate in a one-day continuing education experience they were providing for the Department of Geriatrics, University of South Carolina School of Medicine. My segment was called, "A Day in the Life of a Caregiver". A dear and close friend, Kay O'Connor, drove me to Myrtle Beach for the event. That presentation was the basis of this record. I began with a description

I

of my husband, John Beckler, the best man I ever knew. Here is how I described him:

John, a good student in Benton, Tennessee, was a small town boy who did well. At age fifteen, unbeknownst to anyone, he enrolled himself in Berry School, Rome, Georgia, a school where you could work your way through. He rode a bus to Berry's renowned Gates of Opportunity, carrying with him a footlocker and $50. Completing his under-graduate work at Tennessee Tech in Cookeville, John received his Masters of Science degree from Vanderbilt University, making one B in college, in a one-hour course. John spent thirty-seven years with Eastman Kodak/Eastman Chemical Co., transferring to Columbia in April, 1984. As President of Carolina Eastman Company, he was very active in the area business environment, serving as President of the South Carolina Chamber of Commerce prior to retirement, April 1, 1996. John Beckler was a wonderful husband, father, friend, a great American, a committed Christian. He possessed a warm, appealing personality, a positive attitude toward life, was optimistic, always looking for the good.

These were John's major resources as he began to cope with the dreadful, unrelenting advance of dementia. Our dear friend and neurologist, Dr. William Brannon, told me that as John's considerable resources were depleted the progression of his illness would quicken. So it did.

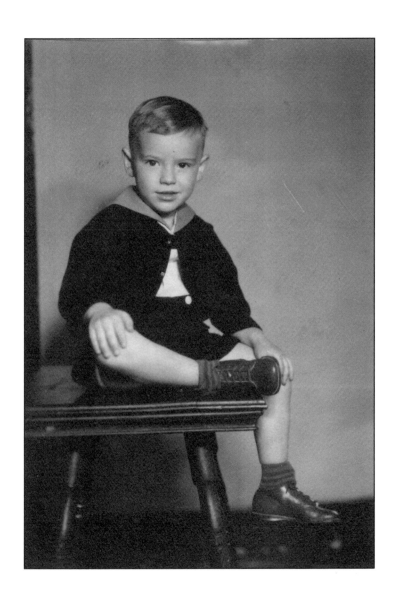

John 1936 (He was four years old.)

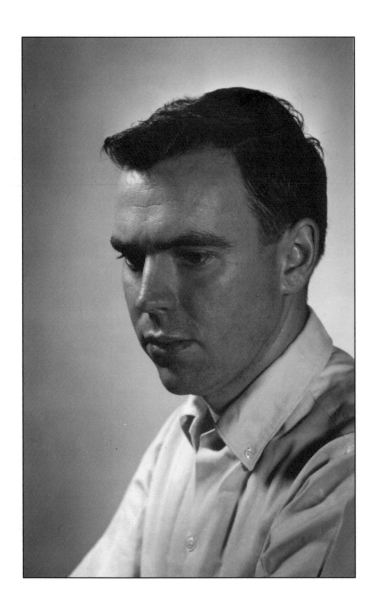

John 1962

THE BEGINNING

"I know I don't listen."

"Why don't you listen?"

"I don't...know."

We both were silent all the way home. Thus, we had stated the primary issue that was to impact the coming years, ultimately to dominate every second of our lives, right to the moment of John's death, September 13, 2010.

Following John's retirement, we soon began to experience problems in meeting away from home for such things as servicing a car, sharing a lunch date, arriving at some agreed-upon location for a movie, dinner, or to consider a possible purchase. I would wait at the appointed place, following the long established wisdom to never, ever leave the designated spot. Time would pass; I, frozen in frustration. "Here you are! Where have you been? I have been looking everywhere for you!" There he would be, that happy voice, the warm greeting, the engaging smile I had loved since we met through mutual friends in the summer of 1955. *Where had I been, indeed!*

The developing crisis in our life came to a head in November, 1996. In the months preceding John's retirement, he really couldn't remember much at home. I had always taken care of things there and just felt he was definitely in the pre-retirement "windingdown" mode and tried to be patient, taking care of even more things for him. I did think he was carrying the "winding down" a bit far when I would have to tell him often as many as three times what our plans were for the evening or weekend. Some of the forgetfulness certainly gave me pause, and I wondered what was happening at work where he had a very good secretary. Eventually some aspects just didn't make sense, but we couldn't really look at anything seriously until retirement.

Following his retirement in April, 1996, several puzzling things were happening:

What should have been a normal adjustment of easing into a more relaxed lifestyle evolved into inertia and lethargy.

He demonstrated an increasing inability to remember daily events and times, to read and interpret data on our family calendar in the kitchen.

He became confused and bewildered over something as simple as meeting me for lunch, meeting me to shop, arranging car repairs, all in locations long familiar and often frequented.

Of major concern to us both, he frequently missed board and committee meetings downtown because of inability to locate offices and buildings he knew quite well.

He became uncertain of notes he now carried in his pocket.

I once called John from the Ford facility where I had waited an hour for him to pick me up. He was home in his pajamas in the late morning when I reached him. Another long wait until he came for me. Driving home, there was no apology, no explanation. How could he since he did not know! On the cold and windy Tuesday night before Thanksgiving, 1996, John left me waiting in a restaurant in Five Points, by this time frantic over what was happening to us. He had decided his note regarding our dinner plans was wrong, discarded it, had gone early and driven around Five Points for about forty-five minutes, left, gone home. Actually, his note had been wrong earlier but we had corrected it. Of course, he had no memory of that.

Now, I have to say, in the terror of that entire evening, life (God) was working to embrace and sustain our family. Our two daughters, their husbands who are like our sons, and our five grandchildren were in route to Columbia for Thanksgiving, coming from three different directions. Some were there by the time I arrived home. My older daughter said she had never seen her father that upset, pacing the floor, saying he had treated me terribly, didn't understand what had happened, just a terrible mix-up. When I arrived home, every light inside was on, every spotlight outside our home was on, and John was rushing down the stairs to meet me. We had a sleepless night. The next morning early, my sweet husband said, "Pat, something is terribly wrong." I said what all good wives say at those moments, "Don't worry. We'll just find out what it is and decide what to do."

By the end of the next week, with the knowledge, encouragement and full support of our children and older "grands", John had had an MRI, was on medication, was scheduled for his first neuropsychological test, and we were adjusting to hearing such words as *dementia, severe memory impairment,* possible *Alzheimer's, "can slow the progression but not prevent or cure",* and *"need to develop coping procedures."*

So began our journey into the great unknown of emotional fragility and deteriorating mental capacity. We began it, as we had done everything else in our, now forty-seven years of marriage, *together.*

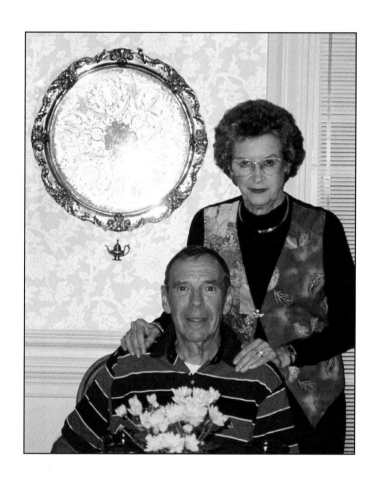

Our dining room,
Oak Brook Drive Columbia, South Carolina

PERSONAL NOTE TO MY SISTERS AND BROTHERS ON A SIMILAR JOURNEY...

If you are not comfortable or interested in reading *our* story, perhaps feel too pressed to even take the time, are more in need of help and guidance or confirmation that you are doing most everything right and/or you are doing most everything that can be done, go quickly to page 59, *Pat's Rules for the Road.* Bottom line...those rules *are* the bottom line.

In reading *Rules* again after many years, I realize how helpful they were for me. Even with my research, you are still "making it up" as you go along, as I did with the *Rules.* Living with dementia was new territory for me. I had no training for losing my husband. I had to create some kind of order in midst of the chaos of the unknown and unexpected so that we could manage and survive in the best way for us all. Thus, I began to develop strategies that became *Pat's Rules.* No day was quite like the day before. Yet there was the consistency of the advancing decline. It was not to be stopped. It had be recognized and endured. I included the

Rules in my talk in 2003, seven years after we began our journey. It helps to learn quickly, confirm what you have discovered, and go forward. You have no other choice. Be compelled to put words to your actions as they become the stepping stones of your journey. Others will follow.

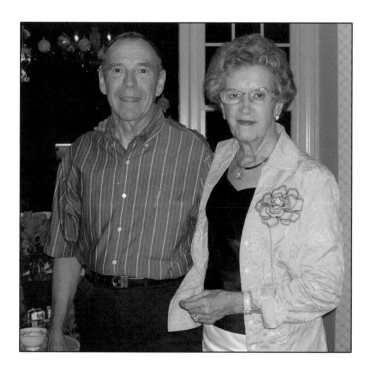

Still on Oak Brook, 2006

"I NEED TO RECONSIDER."

Although John enjoyed travel very much, he perhaps did not have the passion for new places that I seem to have. Thus, in addition to the many trips we made during his vacations, I did many tours "alone on a tour" or, a few times, "alone". This did not present a problem until we realized he could not be left alone. Cheryl suggested that, since my trip of the moment was a Smithsonian tour of the West Indies, he could stay with her with a convenient departure for me from Jacksonville, Florida. Great idea, or so it seemed. When presented to John, he first agreed. Later he said he would go with me to Cheryl's in Waycross, Georgia, return to Columbia, and then back to Waycross again upon my return. Oh, dear, what now? My air schedule was already purchased! Time passed with no resolution until John received a very sweet birthday card from Cheryl. She mentioned how much she hoped to have him visit with her family during my absence. A very touched John Beckler said to me, "I think I need to reconsider." So it was! Thank you, Cheryl.

Thank you, God. It was a splendid trip for me and a meaningful experience for John.

Reflecting on this more than a decade later, I am aware that, at that point, John could still process simple sequential steps in an activity. Driving to Cheryl's home, delivering me to the airport, returning to Columbia, and back to Waycross. I can still feel the momentary relief of his change of heart. It was not to last.

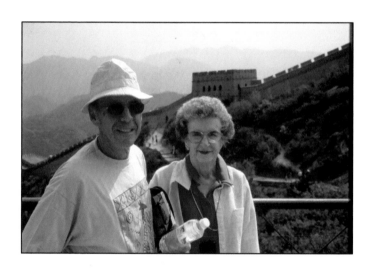

P & J Great Wall China, 2002

"NOW YOU WANT TO DISCUSS IT!"

Not long after John's retirement, we spent a week at DisneyWorld in Orlando. We did all the fun things: rode "It's A Small World" many times and watched the water show from our balcony in the late evening. The last couple of days I wanted us to pinpoint and organize the remaining activities we would be interested in doing. We were inside having a cool drink. I was reading from the Guidebook, questioning John on various things. He was totally uncooperative, shook his head in discomfort and would not engage in the discussion. In frustration, I ceased the attempted dialogue.

Out we went, late morning, into the very warm day. As we walked along, I noted some event that was nearby and asked if he would enjoy that. He said, "Yes." in a very officious, offended and demeaning way, "Yes, I WOULD LIKE to do that SOMETIME," as if I were somehow preventing him. I threw down the Guidebook. "I have tried for thirty minutes to have this discussion with you. NOW, that we are out in the heat, you want to discuss it."

It was not a good day.

When my publisher, Mary Catharine Nelson, read my first draft, she questioned me on how I coped with the everyday happenings as the experiences within this book are often monumental in importance. Like life itself, the significant moments frequently occur in "a normal day", an unimportant day. Often their profound meaning isn't obvious at the time. Perhaps to state again, the *Rules*, as they formed themselves in my mind, helped me to focus with some objectivity and rational thought as my heart was breaking. No one said this would be easy.

"I CANNOT READ THIS BOOK."

In the early days, it was important for me to become as informed as possible on dementia. A good friend gave me a copy of *THE 36-HOUR DAY*, said to be the definitive book of the times. As a life-long "bookaholic" I had always looked to books for entertainment, information, direction, and inspiration. I started that book three times, quickly absorbing the opening chapters of comfort, affirmation, encouragement...all the things I needed at that time. Moving forward, I would engage the sections on coping techniques, the "how-to's", and adjustments to the home environment that would be helpful to the loved one.

Steps!!! We had five flights of steps in our home, three interior flights and two exterior. The book recommended painting each step a different color so the loved one would realize he/she was ascending or descending. Three times I stopped, unable to proceed. I could not go beyond that point. At life's most challenging moments, we desire to be strong, to do what is required to take care of our loved ones. We do have our limits. Our home was decorated in light pastels. To envision the intrusion of bright reds and blues and purples, beautiful though they are, was more than I could accept.

The book I did read and have shared with others was *THE FEARLESS CAREGIVER*, a later definitive book. Ah, yes, that was my book! It put into words before my eyes the principles I was constructing for my new role as Caregiver. (See *Pat's Rules for the Road*, page 59.)

"MARILYN, WE NEED TO TALK."

As close as our family is, the steps on this journey were most often taken by those present on a daily basis. When, of necessity, I changed housekeepers, I did not realize at first it was the beginning of one of God's most tender gifts for me. Marilyn and David Williams were educators, having at least three degrees between them. Deciding to leave the academic world, David pursued his wish to form his own (very meticulous, near perfection) paint and remodeling company. In her quiet time, Marilyn, in surprise, discerned that she should clean houses. Now, really! When I met this poised, soft-spoken, elegant woman, she was only available one day every other week. OK. Let's try that. Over time I was able to increase her days as they became available. Ultimately, Marilyn wrote a beautiful letter to her other clients telling them she felt called to work full time for the Beckler's. During that period I was in and out, often gone during lunch time. As Marilyn spent more time with us, I wondered when the time would come when she and I would experience our first of MANY heart-to-heart talks. Eventually, some question arose and I knew the moment was upon us. "Marilyn, we need to talk." We withdraw to The Painted Room, our guest room dedicated to our granddaughters. I shared our history with the memory deterioration. What a surprise for me to learn that John and Marilyn, when lunching alone, had developed a very consistent pattern. The nice lunch in our kitchen or on our back porch provided the platform for John's sharing his life story—childhood, education, family, career. Marilyn said it took him about thirty minutes, the narrative being a repeat of the day before. She could quote sections from memory. Concluding, he would speak of me, our life together and end with these words, "And, you know, she loves me."

"Yes, John, I do love you...now and forever."

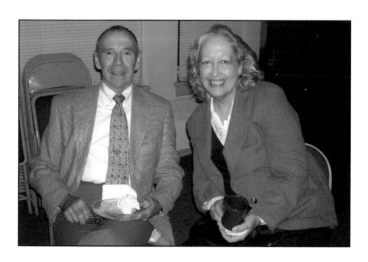

Marilyn and John, around 2003

"WE HAVE TO CHANGE SOME THINGS."

In our very first visit to neurologist, Dr. William Brannon, in early December, 1996, we learned in order to make a formal diagnosis we must develop a history, our consultation with him being our first step. Following an MRI the next week, we soon began periodic testing done by a neuro-psychiatric specialist. These were grueling experiences lasting several hours. We would begin with the two of us having dialogue with the doctor. My primary role was to indicate how accurately John responded to the questions. Some questions were directed at me, especially in the early moments. This seemed to relieve his apprehensions somewhat, and I soon would be excused....to wait...and wonder where we were going. The results of the battery of the tests, along with the doctor's evaluation would be forwarded to me. I always shared these with our daughters.

The sessions were quite exhausting for John. He would appear withdrawn and almost white with fatigue. I usually scheduled them in the morning when he would be at his freshest and then followed with a pleasant lunch in a new or especially enjoyable restaurant. Something of a recovery. We did these tests annually in the early years, then skipped a few years. This time the regression was significant. Stunning. I knew it. John knew it. No pleasant midday meal that day. Neither of us was up to it. I suggested we go home, have a quick lunch and make some decisions. So...sitting there at our kitchen table, I said that I thought we should revise some of our plans. First, I thought that we should abandon our plan for John to supervise construction of a patio home, for which we had already purchased two lots in Turkey Pointe, a small section of WildeWood dedicated to that style living. Second, we would stay in our large home as long as we could, skip the interim "down-sizing" phase, eventually move to a small retirement community at the appropriate time. My real reason for staying where we were was I realized it was long past a good time to move and expect John to make an easy transition into a new and strange setting. In addition, "staying put" would give us the space to hire what help we would need as time went by.

Then, to my great astonishment, John added a third decision. He told me that it was time to examine the ownership of our assets, changing everything that could be put into my name alone. We must meet our financial manager, Bill

Walkup, and our attorney so they could develop the plan and see it through. Then, with tears in his eyes...as well as mine...he handed me his credit cards. This was the wise and courageous man I had been married to for almost fifty years! No wonder I loved you, John Beckler!

It took several months to make the changes, with numerous trips for me back and forth. With each set of papers, I wanted to explain the steps being taken and the signatures—mostly his—required to implement. John wanted no discussion or explanations. Just show him where to sign.

I have always thought the family kitchen was the "power center" of most any home. Discussions held. Decisions made. Lives changed. True at least for the Beckler's. I believe that day was the last significant cognitive activity for my intelligent, caring husband. Assured that I would be taken care of and that our family was protected, he clearly resigned himself to the coming days, months, years ahead. Bless you, John.

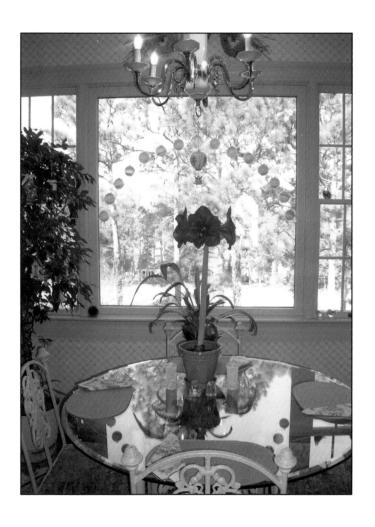

Our Oak Brook Drive kitchen

THE MYSTERY OF THE BRAIN

Given the persistence of the advancing dementia, it is intriguing to contemplate the astonishing "happenings" along the way. Cognitive activity from your loved one is no longer occurring. It would be cruel to all involved to expect it. Yet, there are those unexplainable moments. During one of John's psycho-neurological tests, the doctor showed him three items. First, there was the notepad. Second, there was a glass. Third, there was a ball-point pen. I was told that John struggled with the first two, taking a very disappointing length of time to identify each one. With the third, the doctor expected his slow response to be "a ball-point pen" or just "a pen". Instead, John very quickly, clearly, and with total confidence spoke the multi-syllable chemical compound that composed the particular type of plastic from which the pen was made. It's as if some unseen force within the intricacy of the deteriorating brain is just checking to be sure you are paying attention!

"I DON'T WANT TO BE A DANGER TO OTHERS."

When dementia penetrates a family, every person and every relationship, all traditions and rituals, holidays and visits—everyone and everything feels the impact. The situation is also influenced by the gender of the memory-impaired person. So, in our case, *driving* was a major issue. We had gently moved into the habit of my driving when we were together. John was cooperative, although I think he realized it was strategy on my part, when I suggested driving because "he was tired". I had become increasingly concerned for several months. I burst into tears one evening when he had slammed on the breaks at an intersection, expressing anger at having to stop. But stop he did. Just in time. I said, "John, you are frightening me."

The most alarming experiences would occur at a major intersection on our way to church, namely Jackson Blvd., Devine Street, and a secondary road, the three converging in front of Bojangles.

One Sunday morning I initiated a conversation, calling attention to the hazards of the intersection and said, "John, one day you saved our lives by looking and seeing a woman run a red light in her haste to reach Bojangles. You LOOKED and STOPPED just in time." He seemed to comprehend. As we approached, the light was red. He did slow down briefly; but as the light changed to green, he began moving forward without looking in any direction, saying, "That is the longest light in Columbia." I was sick at heart.

Since, at least at that time, only simulated driving tests were available in Columbia, I believe Senior Primary Care thought John was intelligent enough to possibly pass those, and so they made arrangements for him to be tested in Augusta. There, the road test was a vital segment of the experience. Off we went. To say I was stressed does not provide sufficient understanding of my conflicted state of mind. I thought, if he passed, I was not sure I could continue with the fright of his driving. Yet, I dreaded the impact of his becoming disqualified to drive.

There was a lengthy oral segment as well as written. Then, the road test. He and the examiner, a very pleasant young woman, were gone an hour. I was unable to read. Unable to sit still. I checked in with the counselor at SPC. A torturous period of time. Upon their return, I could see John exit our vehicle. His face looked like a child on Christmas morning! He clearly believed he had done well. The nice lady began her comments in a very positive way. He had done well on the oral and reasonably well on the written. John was delighted. I was breathless. "However, Mr. Beckler, you did not do well on the road. So I must tell you, you must no longer drive."

The stunned, disbelieving, devastated look on John's face was extremely painful to see. Yes, I was the one who wept—almost sick with relief as well as sad beyond words for my sweet husband. No resistance. Sad acceptance. John, the realist.

On our way home we stopped for something to drink. No conversation had occurred at this point. Then, John said. "I don't want to be a danger to others. I want Richard to have my car." Amazing! We had to keep this one-year-old Honda CRV a year for Richard, our only grandson, to reach sixteen. I have a picture of John's handing him the keys, birthday cake clearly visible. How can I recall one of the worst days of my entire life with an element of joy in my heart? The answer is gratitude. Thank you, John, for being the person you were, the husband you were, the grandfather you were.

As of this writing, June 6, 2015, Richard is still driving this aging vehicle with 168,000 miles on it. His parents are providing him a newer means of travel as he departs for a career on the west coast. Go, Richard!! Drive carefully! Don't forget your Papa John!

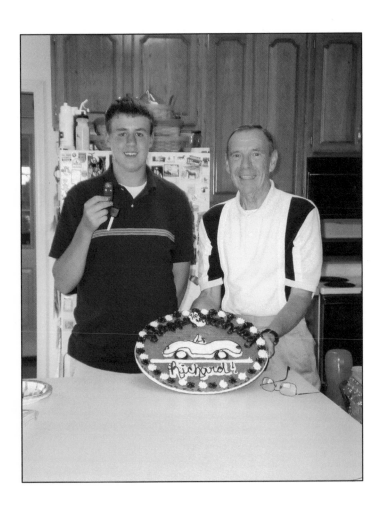

Richard and John, July 3, 2007

"I'M GOING TO UN-COMMIT!"

Oddly enough, there were moments when the chuckles came forth. (Isn't it wonderful that God gave us humor?) There were also times when I felt quite certain my guardian angel gave me the words to change John's behavior or interrupt his activity of the moment.

Obviously not as dangerous as the driving issue, but actually more stressful because it was almost a daily issue, was The Sprinkler System. We had a fairly good size yard and a very complicated irrigation system. We had eight stations with as many as fourteen heads each. John was forever making adjustments as he was constantly moving, adding to, rearranging his plants and shrubs, borders, a small fountain, brick walkway, stone path. You name it. Of course, the time came when his "adjustments" were such that I would have to call our two "yard men" who did the mowing and anything else we needed. (These two gentlemen were actually retired businessmen who enjoyed landscaping and irrigation issues.) Each visit was a minimum of $45.00, not to mention the cost to my emotional wellbeing. At a crucial point one dreadfully hot day, I called the counselor at Senior Primary Care. As John and I stood there in the blazing heat, she talked him through to the moment when he promised me he would never touch the system again. I know that, at the time, he sincerely intended to honor that pledge to me. *The next day* I saw him in the front yard obviously beginning a *major* adjustment. Yes, I went charging out to stop him. No, I was not loving and patient! John asked me why he couldn't continue. I said, because the day before he had committed to leave things alone.

He said, "Well, I'm going to un-commit."

"No, you won't"

"Why not?"

"Because you haven't broken a promise to me in almost fifty years and you are not going to start today!"

He put away his tools and went inside, spent. So was I. He was my John again.

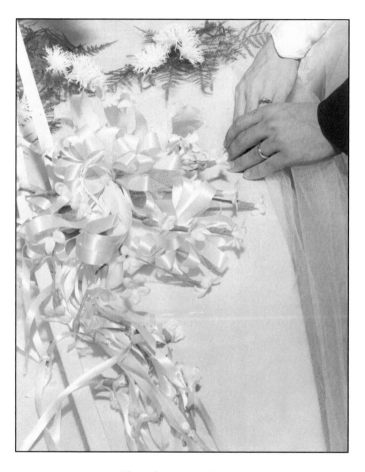

Our wedding day, December 22, 1956

THE POWER OF MUSIC

One of the things I dreaded most was the moment when I would need to withdraw John from his beloved Celebration Choir at Shandon United Methodist Church, our home church since moving to Columbia in 1984. We were very active members in this large downtown congregation, having numerous responsibilities along the way. This new choir was our "second" choir, so to speak, with a simpler repertoire than our Chancel Choir, singing monthly and on special occasions. Although not a choir member, I was a great supporter and had been present when the name was chosen. Many members were especially close friends as well as being J.O.Y. Sunday School classmates. Through the years, "On Eagles Wings" had become their unofficial theme song. Participation had become somewhat difficult for John and was possibly becoming a distraction for the fellows around him. The time came, around 2006 or 2007, when fall rehearsals began, John was not aware that the choir was going forward without him. I wondered if he would realize the change the next Sunday when they sang. I was alarmed when the Order of Worship listed …you guessed it… "On Eagles Wings" as the anthem. When the service began, he stirred a little, realized something was different but not what, gazed intently at the choir up front, appeared more puzzled and bewildered than actually troubled. Time for the anthem. John still did not understand the changed circumstances but knew something was most assuredly altered. As the choir sang that lovely hymn, he became quite agitated, moved around in his seat, was on the verge of speaking. I took his arm on one side and a dear J.O.Y. SS class member took the other. That beautiful music was calling John, and he knew not how to answer.

"THIS IS NOT PHYSICAL. THIS IS VERY EMOTIONAL."

Those of you who knew John Beckler will be astonished to hear that, separate and apart from the driving episodes, I was actually frightened twice. The more serious one is lodged forever in my mind and heart. After a major upset, with angry words spoken, John followed me into the kitchen. He hardly looked like himself. He realized that I had moved to the other side of the island. I was crying. In a cold and unfamiliar voice he said, "This is not physical. This is emotional, very emotional." Dementia at it's worst. The person you know and love is gone.

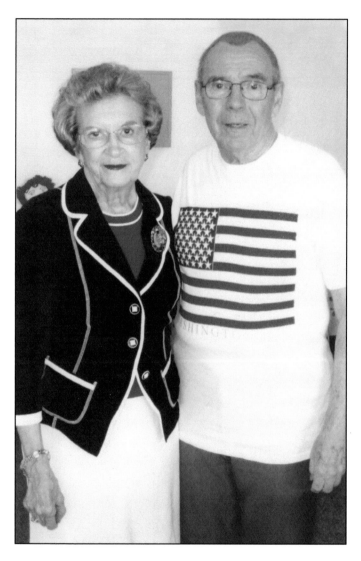

LifeScenes, July 2010
Dementia unit, Wildewood Downs

"TAKE IT AWAY! TAKE IT AWAY!"

As I have written our story, I have been reminded of how close our daughters, Cheryl and Celia, were/still are, even now, five years since John's death. As a part of our record, I have retained copies of many emails, notes, summaries of happenings along the way. First, I needed them to know. Second, it was my responsibility to keep them informed should there come a time when the decisions would be theirs to make.

In early 2005, a very serious issue was developing. I quote the following from an email to my girls, March 3, 2005.

Girls, this is just to keep you updated as I think we pass mile markers.

We had a terrible upset Tuesday afternoon. I went in Daddy's study to find him with notebooks emptied, labels removed on several, stacks of files lying around, a few odds and ends. He was very tense and said there was no need to keep everything so far back and he was getting rid of a lot to make more space.

Stressed his need for space. Actually, there was plenty of room in his spacious study.

I was very upset not knowing what was where and what might have already been destroyed. The most alarming thing was a fax I had sent to Fidelity. It was one sheet by itself just ready to fall into the waste paper basket. On it was a hand-written note to remind me of the important step I have to do each year to activate the annual IRA distributions. If you miss, you don't lose the money but get none that year. After a while Daddy started trying to reassemble the contents, relabeling, somehow coming out with two more notebooks than he had started with. No order. I was almost in tears by this time and your Dad was very angry.

Finally, I brought in some large plastic file boxes in which to place the scattered materials. Several notebooks that were still together had been opened, then closed with the clasps still open so pages were falling out. During that process, John started to hyper-ventilate, waving his hands around and kept saying, "Take it away. Take it away." I told him he needed to rest so he actually went to bed until I woke him for dinner. I haven't had the heart to start even thinking about going through and getting things back in order. It is all right there on the king bed in the adjacent bedroom, but out of sight of the doorway. Sometime during that night, it seemed to me that we had passed some kind of marker as normal adult discussions are just about a thing of the past. It upsets me terribly when he promises me he won't do something ever, ever again when I know he will and can't help it. The marker is to avoid explanations and having discussions expecting some understanding. Also, for the first time- almost to start hiding and such.

It has been important to me to avoid deceiving him, and certainly not to trick him. I need to think of secrecy and deception as actually protection from harm of various kinds.

Sorry to bring such news, but this is where we are.

Love you both more than I can say,

MOM

The storage issue was solved by arranging a stacked filing cabinet inside a closet convenient to my work space but situated behind some clothing. Yes, I kept the drawers locked. I needed to be The Fearless Caregiver. I don't believe John ever thought again of where everything had gone or questioned where it all might be now. Another closing.

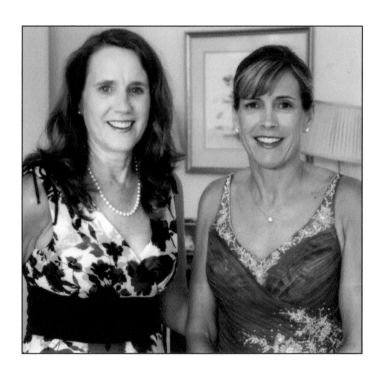

My daughters Celia and Cheryl

JOHN'S LIGHT HOUSE - 2006

When my sweet husband, John, presented me with this watercolor of a light house, I was so touched. I knew it had to be placed where we would see it often. It hung in our kitchen near our table. We, at least I, looked at it often as we shared our meals.

We all understand that lighthouses were originally built to give illumination so that those at sea could find their way to shore even in the deepest dark of night. Many paintings we see of lighthouses are tranquil seaside images with lots of blue sky and water. Others are dark and foreboding with the focal point being that small but vivid light, a beacon for the lost or searching. John's rendering is in dramatic pinks, blues and golds. Life is something like those paintings. Sometimes things are quiet and good and all we would want life to be. At other times, the way seems dark and we search for meaning, understanding, and direction. I still have this painting. It is hanging in my sitting room here at Wildewood Downs. It is a sweet memory of John and a meaningful symbol of our experience with dementia.

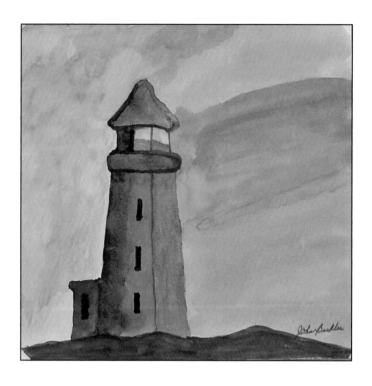

John's Light House, 2006

John's painting was a result of a series of watercolor classes given by our dear friend, Bonnie Mullis. Bonnie wanted to do something for us. As a gifted artist, she offered the classes. Just recently, as I was finishing this book, Bonnie shared an experience similar to Marilyn's—John's life story became a part of their painting sessions. Toward the end, Bonnie mentioned she had never known what my dad, Brandon Lewis, had done for a living. John thought a moment and then said, "He was a Superintendent of Schools." No, John, that's what your father did! My Dad was an attorney, was the Clerk of the Federal Court in Nashville, Tennessee. What kind of a mixup is that? A touching one! Since John never knew his own father, and was very close to mine, it made sense in John's confused mind!

"ARE YOU OVER THERE IN OUR LITTLE HOUSE?"

Dr. Bill Brannon had told me that in a certain number of years I would need to be thinking of a facility for John. He was absolutely on target. Dear friend, Polly Judd, called me one day to say Wildewood Downs was open to putting two lots together so that a larger home could be constructed. I came the next day. This retirement community was within two miles of our home of 21 years. The biggest advantage was the various levels of care provided which would be available to us as we needed them. Our new home, half the size of the one we were in, was built in a few months. We moved in on July 3, 2008. John 's decline, now accelerating, was confirmation that our move had been the appropriate decision. He lived at home with me for almost two years. We moved him into LifeScenes, the dementia unit, March 30, 2010. Dr. Margaret Matthews, our Senior Primary Care physician, told me that John was "so ready" for the limited environment, his adjustment would be quite easy. No more decisions to be made. No more uncertainties or new situations. Everything done for him. The day we moved him, he clearly was puzzled but could not formulate the question, which I knew was, "Why am I here?". I told him that he had medical problems we could no longer take care of at home. He nodded, smiled and said, "You are over there in our little house?" He DID know where I was! His easy adjustment had taken place.

LifeScenes is actually structurally attached to the Wildewood Downs Club House so it was a quick walk from the dining room to see John, a lock-down section with coded entry. Most days I went twice. During his five months there he was never uncomfortable, agitated or troubled in any way. Thank you, Wildewood Downs.

In the fall, 2010, John was taken to Palmetto Health Richland. His body was shutting down. After eleven days, he was returned to Wildewood Downs Skilled Care. I was there when he was carefully rolled down from the vehicle. We had eye-contact the entire time. Strong contact but with no facial change from John. I believe that was the last moment he recognized me. Our last moment as two people who loved each other and were saying good-bye. We believe he suffered a stroke within that first day there. He was on oxygen from then on, did not eat or respond to any of us, just lay there with eyes open, gazing at nothing. He died the evening of September 13, 2010.

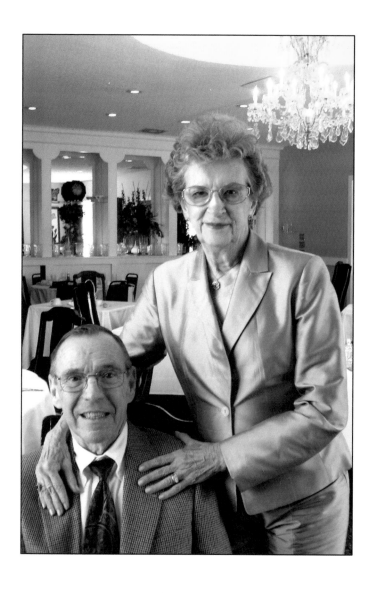

John's last Easter, 2010

MY CHRISTMAS CARD 2010

For many years, I had made our annual Christmas greeting composed of a newsy letter and including photos of our immediate family. Following John's death, our friends received the message:

As most of you know, the angels came for John September 13. He had been in Columbia Heart 11 days and back here in Wildewood Downs Skilled Care Unit for 5 days. We knew several days in advance what was coming and it did. We had a beautiful service of celebration of his life on September 18. I am so grateful to our two daughters (Celia was actually here when it happened) for their constant attention and presence those last days and following. I am also so proud of our whole family during this time and especially for Cheryl, Elizabeth and Richard who spoke at the service. John had been in LifeScenes, the dementia unit here at WD since March 30. Having these levels of care was the primary reason we moved here two years ago. I am in our house we built, feel safe, enjoy new but close friends, and am able to continue with most of the things I have done for years.

Even with this sadness, the great joy of this year has been the birth of our first great-granddaughter, Makayla Monroe Colberg, June 2. John never saw her, did not understand what I was telling him; but she has his genes and hopefully will have his capacity for love, intelligence, compassion, and deep faith.

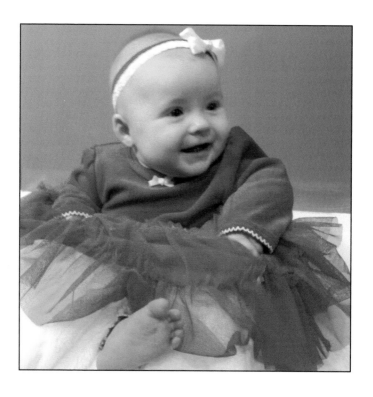

Makayla's first Christmas

"SOMETHING GOD ALONE CAN SEE"

As we began to consider what might be a fitting memorial for John, sculpture seemed a possibility. Not only was sculpture his favorite art form, the growing collection of original art at Shandon United Methodist Church did not, at that point, include sculpture. I had been very much involved in the Music and Arts Ministry for several years. Becoming familiar with the kinetic work of Lyman Whitaker, I watched his creations online, turning, turning. Too many to choose just one. I believe it was dear friend, Jean Hein, who suggested three pieces to correspond with the three verses of John's favorite hymn, "Hymn of Promise" by contemporary composer, Natalie Sleeth. They now reside within the Shandon United Methodist Memorial Garden, very near our niche. On the day of our dedication of the sculptures, several members of our family were joined by J.O.Y. Sunday School class members. Rev. Julie Songer-Belman did a lovely job with the dedication. Yes, the Celebration Choir sang "On Eagles Wings". Both of these beautiful hymns had been sung at our service to celebrate John's life the previous September. The sculptures are never completely still although they sometimes appear that way. Unseen, as is the work of the Holy Spirit, the gentlest of breezes can cause almost imperceptible movement of these amazingly engineered beauties. I am touched by the many comments that I continue to hear. I often stop when I happen to be going by as members or visitors quietly open the gate to venture in. The words of the hymn are available on a brass plaque at the feet of the three pieces.

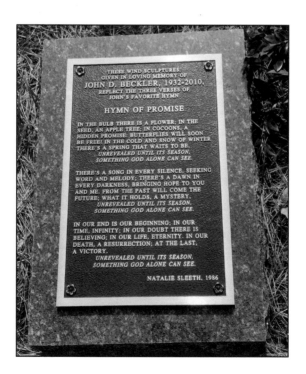

Patricia L. Beckler

Hymn of Promise

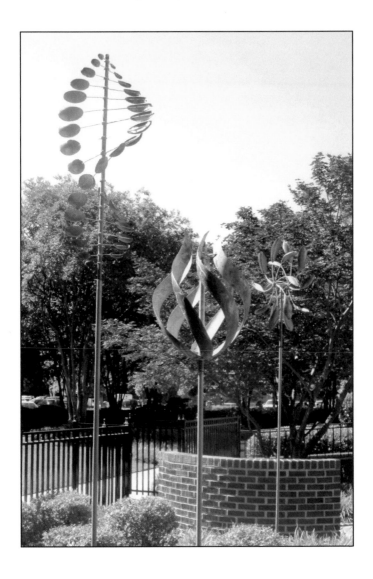

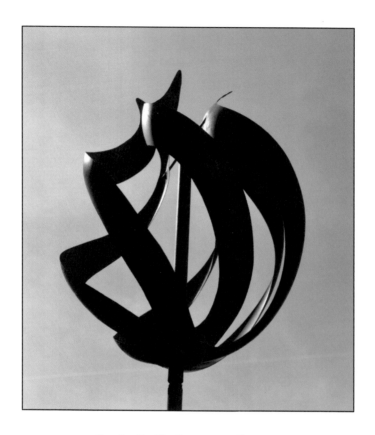

In the bulb there is a flower;
in the seed, an apple tree;
in cocoons, a hidden promise;
butterflies will soon be free!
In the cold and snow of winter
there's a spring that waits to be,
unrevealed until its season,
something God alone can see.

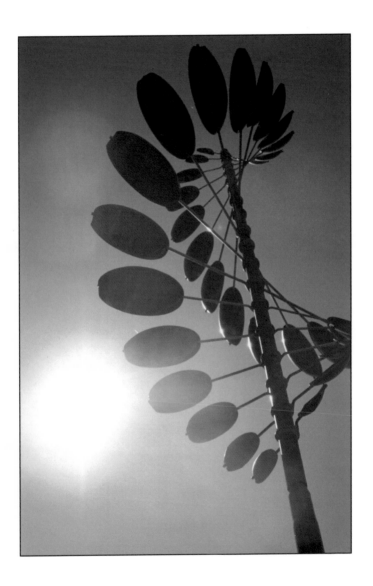

There's a song in every silence,
seeking word and melody;
there's a dawn in every darkness,
bringing hope to you and me.
From the past will come the future;
what it holds, a mystery,
unrevealed until its season,
something God alone can see.

Patricia L. Beckler

In our end is our beginning;
in our time, infinity;
in our doubt there is believing;
in our life, eternity.
In our death, a resurrection;
at the last, a victory,
unrevealed until its season,
something God alone can see.

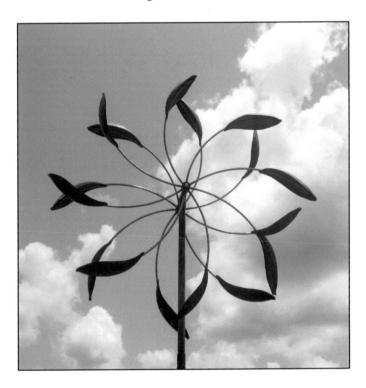

Hymn of Promise, By Natalie Sleeth
in The United Methodist Hymnal, 1998, page 70.

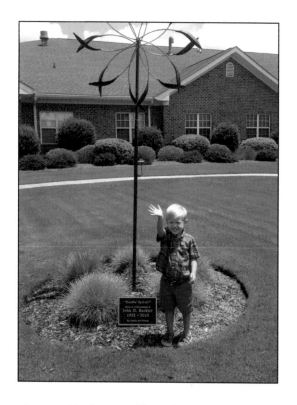

Jamison Pridgen, Wildewood Downs courtyard

We also placed the double spinner (verse three) in the courtyard at Wildewood Downs. Visible from the four surrounding buildings, I have received many calls of inquiry and appreciation from residents who live over in our "medical side", as well as from their family members and visitors. It is illuminated at night.

CONCLUSION:

As our lives were being turned upside down, it was always very important to me that I maintain the element of integrity in all my decisions, adjustments, and arrangements. It still is. I wished to be faithful to our long marriage and relationship, to our wedding vows. I believe I was able to do that. I hope I did.

Good-bye, John Beckler. I love you Now and Forever!

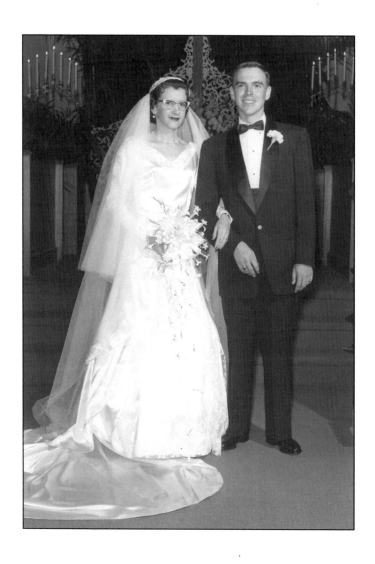

Wedding December 22, 1956

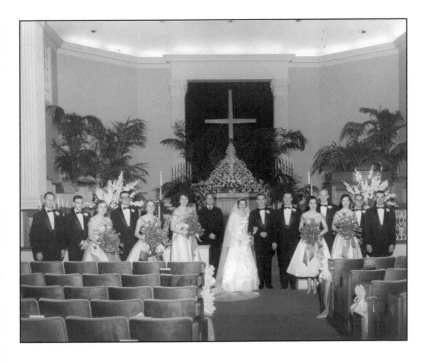

PAT'S RULES FOR THE ROAD

Some people believe that women are born with the nurturing instinct. Others believe that for most of us, life expects us and trains us to be care-givers. Thus, we are ready when care-giving roles come our way. But *there is care-giving and there is care-giving.* As the major care-giver for my mother, I accepted the role reversal from child to parent. As more and more caregiving is required for your spouse, you are losing the care, love and protection that have been yours from this loved one. Simultaneously, you are needing to provide more and more of those precious qualities to that person, in my case, my loving husband. Supply and demand don't balance at either end. So...what are the *Rules for the Road?*

**You had better love this person A LOT. Duty and responsibility will sustain only so long with this type situation. It just carries too much potential stress.

**Educate yourself as soon as possible on the Do's and Don't. It will save heartache, frustration and guilt. Such as: Don't argue, divert. Don't explain, keep things simple. I have validated those things many times!

**Don't wait too long to provide or arrange for help with chores and activities. Resistance from the loved one does not always mean you are pushing too fast. Relief will sometimes emerge and be quite obvious even if not outwardly acknowledged. The "Well Person" makes the decisions, not the "Sick Person". *Read THE FEARLESS CAREGIVER.*

**Have the courage to resist being paralyzed by love for the person. Tough love is not easy. (See previous statement.)

**Remember, sometimes the easiest or best thing for you is also best for the loved one. Don't be intimidated by fear of guilt.

**Try hard to know the difference between what's harmful for the person and what might be just inconvenient or a nuisance to you.

**Make a priority of your own health and well being. *Become* "the fearless care-giver."

** Accept help from others. If someone else can do certain things, let them. (This one might take some work.)

**Expect your priorities to change. At first, I thought the worst thing that could happen to me would be for John to forget me. That would be the worst thing for me. The worst thing *for our family* would be for something to happen to ME, and our daughters would have to step in. Neither John nor I would want that to happen. They would do it, of course. Have no doubt of that.

**Some side issues that are really major issues:

❖ Struggles of guilt-Perhaps it's not such a bad thing that fear of guilt quite often makes us do the right thing. I think that guilt comes from lack of patience, overlooking something, being preoccupied with other matters, just generally not putting the loved-one first. Acknowledge that guilt feelings will come but determine that they will not overwhelm you. Care-givers must function as rational, objective, realistic persons. Nothing will ever be the same again.

❖ Anger-his and hers. Anger is going to happen. *John's*—Confusion and change, fear and uncertainty, inability to assess a situation such as in a restaurant or shopping, my needing to get him to do something he didn't want to do. By nature, John's anger was short-lived, and I learned all kinds of ways to diffuse. *Mine*— when he fakes to avoid the issue of not remembering. It dominates our life so let's be real about it.

❖ Depression/futility of process—One of my greatest concerns because of the fact that, although he was not prone to depression and did not demonstrate it, his father suffered from depression and committed suicide when John was four years old. Thus I couldn't help but watch for signs of depression. The doctors were vigilant in their search. As for me—I had my sad moments. I could be upset, frustrated for brief periods of time, but stress was more familiar to me than a sense of hopelessness. When I couldn't think of anything to actually DO to change the situation, I would have a brief moment of despair. There were times, even with all the help and support I had, when it was just up to me and me alone. It's like childbirth-hospital, doctors, nurses, husband around, there comes a time when it's JUST YOU. At that time, I would feel alone but would know that I was never completely alone. I have a very strong faith and DO know I'm not ever ALL ALONE.

❖ The future—Seek good advice about what lies ahead. Prepare as much as possible. Still, with dementia, surprises are constant.

❖ Loss of friend/companion/loving husband. That is what this book is about.

❖ Struggle of social interactions—John became quieter and quieter. For a while, after he ceased to have sustained interest in extended conversation, he would interrupt or interject some memory from the past. Our best friends heard some things many, many times. Then he started saying— "Have they heard thus-and-so?" Ultimately, he smiled and listened but said little. He loved for us to entertain, always liked to have people in our home, but just got quieter and quieter. We continued with most of our social life in tact but buffets, receptions, and drop-in affairs became a challenge for him. At home, he had abandoned his favorite hobby, the yard. He spent most of his time in his chair, watching TV (not absorbing) or reading (not really).

❖ Retain and be grateful for sweet memories of the past. Yes, they are bittersweet, but they are yours to keep. Remember your loved one as he/she used to be.

❖ *Pray a lot* and always know you are not alone.

Family at John's service, Left to right:

Emily and Jason Pridgen, married May 31, 2008.
Now parents of Jamison Neil, born April 20, 2011,
and Madison Monroe, born March 4, 2015.

Elizabeth Monroe, now married to Matthew Grantham,
December 17, 2011.
Parents of Mason James, born October 15, 2013.

Brandon and Ellen Colberg, married June 3, 2006.
Parents of Makayla Monroe (pictured) born, June 2, 2010,
and Nora Madison, born July 12, 2013.

Moi and Cheryl Monroe, married September 8, 1979.

Pat

Celia and Eddie Johnson, married April 14, 1984.
Richard Edward 111, born July 3, 1989,
and Rachel Emily, born October 23, 1992.

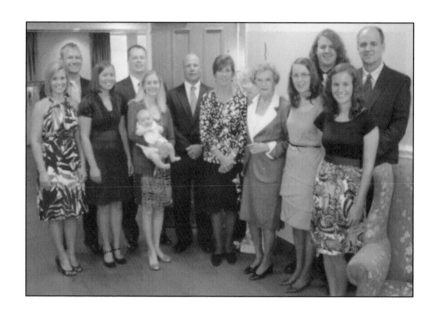

Our family, day of John's service September 18, 2010
Thank you, sweet family, for being there for me!

CPSIA information can be obtained at www.ICGtesting.com
Printed in the USA
LVIW01n1219040116
469016LV00001B/1